Colc

Life's first food

The ultimate anti-aging, immune boosting and weight loss supplement

Daniel G. Clark MD
Kaye Wyatt and David Coory

ZEALAND PUBLISHING HOUSE LTD
Tauranga, New Zealand.

First published   Mar 1996 by CNR Publications,
                Salt Lake City, Utah.
Reprinted   July 1996
Reprinted   Feb   1998
Reprinted   Aug 1998
Revised and reprinted April 2010 by Zealand Publishing House, Tauranga, New Zealand with kind permission of Douglas Wyatt. Director, Center for Nutritional Research (CNR), Sedona, Arizona.
CNR website: www.icnr.org
Thanks also to CNR for updated colostrum information.

This new edition has been revised and updated by health researcher David Coory, author of the book *"Stay Healthy by Supplying What's Lacking in Your Diet"*.

Further copies of this book can be obtained by contacting:
Zealand Publishing House Ltd (trading as Health House)
Private Bag 12029, Tauranga, New Zealand.

Phone   0800 140-141 (NZ only) or International +64 3 520-8103
Fax   0800 140-142 (NZ only) or International +64 7 543-0493
Internet www.healthhouse.co.nz

ISBN 0-908850-43-3

CONTENTS

Colostrum's healing power
Get ready for an
eye opening experience

When a mother gives birth to her offspring, her mammary glands provide life-supporting hormones and disease-fighting antibodies that she has acquired throughout her lifetime.

Her body concentrates these factors into a special pre-milk, growth-supporting and immune fluid called colostrum.

A mother produces this colostrum only during the first 24 to 48 hours after giving birth.

Colostrum a perfect combination for the future health of the newborn

Colostrum is a perfect combination of friendly intestinal microflora, disease antibodies called Immune Factors (or immunoglobulins) and hormones called Growth Factors.

All of these provide immunity to the newborn against future viruses, bacteria, allergens and toxins, and they also provide nourishment for rapid, healthy growth.

The most important meal in our life

The Immune Factors in colostrum, along with desirable acidophilus microflora, 'jump start' the immune and digestive functions in the gut and prevent the development of intestinal and other infections.

The Growth Factors in colostrum help the newborn to grow healthily and to heal quickly if injured.

Colostrum is so important to newborn animals, that most simply die without it.

As it is with animals, so it is with humans, colostrum transmits disease immunity and stimulates healthy, normal growth.

It is known that colostrum triggers at least 50 processes in a newborn that provide lasting benefits, some for a lifetime.

Quite simply, it is the most important meal of our life. It is also the most important food supplement we can get as an adult.

It is the only food supplement with power to destroy viruses.

Cow colostrum virtually identical to human colostrum, but richer

Cow colostrum (or bovine colostrum as it is technically known) is virtually identical to that of humans, but far richer. It contains a much higher percentage of the beneficial Immune Factor antibodies called immunoglobulins and also the hormonal Growth Factors.

Huge number of health benefits for humans

This makes cow colostrum of great benefit to the health of humans. These benefits range from greatly enhanced immunity, to improvement in physical fitness, muscle growth, and rapid healing.

As we age, or become weakened from illness, our body produces less and less of the Immune Factors and Growth Factors we need to fight disease and to heal ourselves rapidly.

Colostrum can restore these life-supporting factors, in perfect combinations. We can increase our longevity, boost our immune system to heal disease and enhance our overall quality of life.

All disease immune related

All disease is immune related. Disease is the result of an under-active or over-active immune system.

Heart disease, cancer, allergies, infections, diabetes, auto-immune disease, ulcers and even aging, are all immune related.

Toxic build-ups in our body and nutritional deficiencies, destroy our immune system.

The face of our planet has changed in just a few generations. Much of our food is now chemically altered and laced with preservatives and antibiotics. Due to the mineral depletion of our topsoil, millions suffer malnutrition from nutrient-poor food.

Colostrum has unprecedented human immune and body cell repair benefits

However, there is a great hope. Hold onto your seats. Get ready for an eye opening experience into the truth, concerning a product some have called the *'discovery of our time'*.

A rediscovery actually. Colostrum has been used successfully throughout history by numerous cultures in the world.

Read and benefit from the research of some of the world's most famous universities, hospitals and medical clinics.

See for yourself colostrum's unprecedented immune and body repair benefits.

My story
by Kaye Wyatt
co-author of this book

That evening, Mother Nature was giving one of her finest performances. She calmed the breeze and brought forth all of summer's wondrous fragrances and sounds, during one of Salt Lake City's spectacular sunsets.

I was sitting next to my husband Doug on our deck that overlooks the valley. I realised that even after all these years, he still had the power to make my heart skip a beat.

I closed my eyes and thought of all the special people who touch my life – a mother I adore, a supportive brother and sister, three almost perfect children, and five perfect grandchildren.

My husband Doug and I have always had the ability to know what the other was thinking at any given moment. So it was no surprise that when my tears welled up, I saw them mirrored in the eyes of my husband.

I've always held the belief that any problem I encounter in life will eventually work out for the best. No matter how hopeless it appears. This evening however, my hope was dissipating. My belief was being challenged. My immune system was losing its fight against continual bacterial and viral infections. I was dying. There would be no *'happy ever after'* for us.

My difficult childhood

My entrance into this world was precarious. My mother barely made it to the hospital in time. Nevertheless, my parents were thrilled. After having a boy first, they now had a little girl.

But their elation was shattered after they brought me home from the hospital. It seemed like I was allergic to this world. During that first month of my life, my breathing became increasingly more erratic and laboured. They realised I was in serious trouble. There was no sleep for my mother as she lay constantly by my side, clutching my hand.

Then for a short time, I stopped breathing altogether and turned blue. My parents insisted on an answer from the doctor.

The medical treatment for my respiratory distress at that time was heavy radiation of the thymus gland. I can't imagine they didn't know that the thymus gland is the master controller of the immune system.

As the years progressed, so did my allergies. I was very allergic to cow's milk, so my parents had to drive long distances to farms for goat's milk. To make sure they would get enough to last a couple of days, they had to get up at the crack of dawn and find it before everyone else did.

Unending asthma, hives and eczema

Despite all of my parent's efforts to keep me away from known allergens, I was continually struggling with asthma, hives and eczema.

I vividly recall vacations that I should have been too young to remember. My memory is of bathrooms in motels, and feelings of panic, due to my serious asthma attacks, reinforced by my parent's anxiety. Waiting for steam from the shower to give me back my breath.

Drugs and cortisone shots

When I was older, they were able to control the severity of my asthma attacks with drugs and cortisone shots.

The stage was now set for the fight of my life. A fight for survival, due to a radiation-weakened immune system and drugs that proved to be deadly boomerangs.

Antibiotics almost every month

After the birth of my third child, my asthma seemed to lessen, but bacterial and viral infections in my bronchioles and lungs took its place.

I was teaching junior high school. Between the germs that my children brought home, and the germs I picked up at school, I remember taking a course of antibiotics almost every month.

When I think back to that time of my life, I should have questioned why my body was having more difficulty with illness and healing than other people.

I came home looking like a skeleton

When I was 25, I had a partial hysterectomy. Three weeks later, I was still in the hospital with infection and recurring hemorrhaging.

I came home looking like a skeleton. It took months, with my mother's help, to get me back on my feet.

Endless dental troubles

A couple of years after that, I had my wisdom teeth removed. I remember my dentist telling me how rare it was for a person to have a dry socket, so I needn't worry about infection. But the dry sockets took months to heal. I remember the pain being unbearable. He assured me that it couldn't happen again.

With me it could, and did.

About 10 years ago, I finally reached the point where I was unable to work because of constant dental surgeries and associated infections.

Of course, more antibiotics were called for.

Root canal surgeries could not be done the traditional way, they had to go through the gums, because my roots had calcified. My dentist said he thought it had something to do with my body's inability to heal.

After that, as much as I needed to work, and as much as I wanted to work, I couldn't. I would only last a one or two hours each morning. Then my temperature would soar and I would collapse in bed.

The nuisance of accompanying fever blisters was unending.

I move to natural antibiotics

About this time, because I needed two or three antibiotics in a row to control an infection, Doug told me there would be no more antibiotics.

His mother had used herbs for healing, since he was a child. He said that from this day forward, I would use the natural antibiotics Echinacea and Goldenseal. As they didn't destroy the body.

I don't remember one day not feeling sick

Life was even more difficult from that point on, for both Doug and I. We could never plan to do anything. A vacation, a day's adventure, or even an evening out.

Eventually I would force myself to go out for a day, or an evening with my husband. However, within a very short time my rising fever would prevent any enjoyment for me, and I would just want to be home in bed. For those 10 years, I don't remember even one day, not feeling sick.

During that time, Doug and I investigated everything that might possibly lead to my healing. I enrolled in nutrition classes at the university. He purchased health-related cook books (his hobby is cooking). Every week we would visit the library and end up bringing home stacks of books.

We found the mind-body connection to be the most promising. I had the honour of working with one of the finest hypnotherapists in the world, Ormond McGill. I feel that his work made it possible for me to survive until I found colostrum.

Money wasted on 'miracle cures'

And of course, like so many people with chronic sickness, we wasted a lot of time and money on miracle cures. This was the reason I refused to try colostrum. I felt that anything that made so many promises, could not possibly be true.

Doug tells me not to give up hope

As the brilliance of the Salt Lake City sunset faded, and with tears in his eyes, Doug took my hand and asked me not to give up hope.

This was my stage of life at the beginning of this story.

I reluctantly try colostrum

Two days later, Doug brought home a jar of bovine colostrum that he had purchased from a naturopathic doctor. It cost him $160. He was excited as he told me about the Immune and Growth Factors in colostrum.

But I felt that this was money we could ill afford to spend, especially on another disappointment. I told him that the last thing I needed right now were Growth Factors to make my feet grow bigger. Growth Factors don't do that of course.

I didn't take the colostrum.

Two days later I fell and seriously injured my knee. I began haemorrhaging blood into my kneecap. We immediately went to the emergency clinic, where they put my leg in a Velcro cast. They told me to stay off it, and keep it elevated for two weeks.

When I got home, I was trembling with pain. I said to Doug, "Okay, I'm ready to take your medicine". (Although that's not quite how I said it.) I took a heaped tablespoonful of the colostrum with some water.

At first I couldn't get to sleep that night with the cast on my leg. So Doug helped me take it off.

The beginning of my new life

The next morning, Doug was the first one up. He was reading the newspaper when I arose from bed and went into the kitchen to pour myself some juice.

He looked at me strangely and kept repeating my name. It took me a moment before I realised that I was standing pain free, on a leg that I couldn't put any weight on the evening before.

I pulled up my nightgown and looked down at my knee. It showed no sign that anything had ever happened to it.

This was the beginning of a new life for me. Two days later, my usual high temperature dropped to normal. It never rose again.

Also, no more fever blisters.

There were many, many changes in my body, which I discovered later from research articles, were attributable to the colostrum.

My toenails begin growing pink and healthy

Later on, I noticed that my toenails were now beginning to grow pink and healthy. Before colostrum, the doctor was considering removing them, because of an advanced fungus, the result of years of antibiotic use.

My depression disappears

Two years ago, my doctor tested me for Serotonin uptake, because I was having episodes of severe depression. He told me that my tests were the worst he'd ever seen. He said that people in my condition were known, in a split second, to drive off a cliff. I didn't realise I was that bad.

The antidepressants prescribed for me created frightening side effects and did not help.

When I started taking colostrum, I had no idea that it would help with the depression. However, within a very short time, I felt as if a huge weight had been removed. Life was beautiful and meaningful.

I had to find out if it was the colostrum. So I purposely stopped taking any for a few days.

It was definitely the colostrum. While I was not taking it, I would wake up each morning with the intention to accomplish a lot that day. But my good intentions and the energy to carry them through, fizzled out before I even began.

My thinking wasn't as clear, and according to one of my friends, I was no longer my new, happy self. She said after talking to me on the telephone for a few minutes, "You've stopped taking your colostrum, haven't you?"

My dentist couldn't believe his eyes

I had another pleasant surprise. The naturopathic doctor that introduced us to colostrum told me that it might help my gingivitis. My dentist had said that I might have to consider gum surgery, as the gingivitis was so advanced.

I had very sensitive teeth and sore and bleeding gums.

So for two weeks I packed my gums with powdered colostrum, every evening. That's all it took.

On the next visit, my dentist couldn't believe his eyes. I showed no signs of gingivitis. He is now recommending colostrum to all of his patients.

Immediate improvement in bowel health

Bowel health is of critical importance. This can be something we don't even talk about to ourselves. I realise now, how seriously ill I was in this area before colostrum.

I feel that bowel health is an area that people who begin taking colostrum, will notice a difference immediately. It will be most beneficial for their health.

Severe 'purple' sprain heals in two days

A word of warning. If you take colostrum, you may never get any sympathy again.

Doug went out of town on business for a few days. I tripped on a chair leg and seriously sprained my big toe. It swelled up and turned purple, clear up to my ankle.

My neighbour, who is a nurse, looked at my foot and said I probably wouldn't be able to wear a shoe for at least a month.

How was I going to pick up my husband, the day after tomorrow at the airport?

Miraculously, I walked the whole length of the airport to meet his plane. No pain. No swelling. No discolouration, and no sympathy.

My immune system strengthened more than I ever believed possible

I recently went to stay a week with my daughter who lives in a small town in Wyoming. I was greeted with hugs and kisses by all of her family.

I had been told a year ago, that if I got pneumonia again, I could not count on antibiotics to help. Within days, I started getting nervous. Everyone in my daughter's family suddenly became very sick. They had bad colds and complained of raw, sore throats. One was even taken to hospital with pneumonia.

Some of my food choices in the first few days of my vacation had not been the best for my immune system. We ate doughnuts for breakfast, went swimming in the outdoor hot springs pool in freezing temperatures, and I ate more of the kind of junk food you know you shouldn't eat.

This would certainly be the ultimate test for colostrum. I had been taking colostrum now for almost eight months.

A doctor explained to me that sometimes it takes two or more months for colostrum to strengthen an immune system as weak as mine.

It strengthened mine more than I ever imagined possible. My

daughter and I got the sniffles for about an hour one morning and that was it. My daughter also takes colostrum.

That was the first time in my life that my immune system won.

The lifeguard asked my daughter if I was her sister

The next day when I went swimming with my daughter at the local hot springs, I received an unexpected compliment. I had forgotten to bring my bathing suit on the vacation and had to borrow one from her. (It would have to be a bikini.) The cute, young lifeguard at the pool was actually flirting with me. He asked my daughter if I was her sister.

I have always been slender. However since I had children I had carried unwanted weight around my waist. It has now all gone and I am able to wear the same size jeans I wore in my early 20's.

My muscles are toned, with no trace of cellulite, and my varicose veins have disappeared. The only exercise I've had time for, in the last eight months is walking my dog.

My hair is finally healthy. It is shiny and all the same length, which was impossible before, with breakage and split ends.

I don't know if it's the radiance of health and feeling on top of the world, or the outward physical changes. But everybody I know who has taken colostrum for at least two months, looks shockingly younger.

Throughout history, we have been searching for the fountain of youth. I think the search may be over.

Once dying dog now playfully acting like a puppy

I've talked with so many people about how colostrum has dramatically changed their lives. One of my favourite stories is from a mother, who had suffered crippling arthritis for years. Colostrum made it possible for her to walk again, and to resume the hobbies she loves, without pain.

Several months ago, her vet recommended that they put their family dog to sleep, as he was showing signs of heart failure. He was listless, barely eating, and his body was bloating. She and her grown children were distraught.

In desperation, she sprinkled colostrum on what little food he would eat. Within days the dog had his appetite back. His bloating had disappeared and he was playfully acting like a puppy.

She recently said to me, *"His coat is shiny again and he is so active he seems to have forgotten his age"*. She also said, *"He's always acts as if he's smiling"*.

Her children were so impressed at the changes in the dog, they've all started taking colostrum too.

Colostrum really works

Colostrum works. It really works.

But remember, each one of us is unique in regard to age, weight, progression of illness and lifestyle. We each require more, or less colostrum. I've found that my body needs more colostrum than most people.

I understand colostrum has no drug interactions and is completely safe at any level, with no side effects.

How much should you take?

I take three 500mg capsules first thing in the morning on an empty stomach, and again in the afternoon. You need to work with your own body and let it tell you what you need.

But most of all, please be patient. Although colostrum begins it's healing and cell repair immediately, it may have a lot of work to do.

Thanks to Dr Daniel Clark MD

I want to thank all the people who have put so much of their time and effort into gathering information, researching and writing, to bring colostrum to the public's awareness.

I especially want to thank Dr Dan Clark, MD, for stepping up and caring enough to write about this remarkable rediscovery.

I hear of so many children and adults today who are suffering from life-threatening diseases. Dr. Clark has taken us one step closer to reach out to these people, and ask them not to give up hope for a new life.

Colostrum's Transfer Factors

Colostrum works because of its powerful Transfer Factors.

The term 'Transfer Factor' means that the immune antibodies and growth hormones in colostrum, can be orally transferred (via the mouth and the digestive system) from one mammal to another and still function as Nature intended.

The two main types of transfer factors in colostrum are Immune Factors (antibodies to kill bacteria and viruses) and Growth Factors (hormones to promote youthful growth and healing).

These Immune Factors and Growth Factors are tiny protein-like substances, essential to immunity, growth and healing in newborn mammals. They also work well with adult mammals, including humans.

Bovine (cow) colostrum is far richer in these numerous transfer factors than human colostrum, and they can be fully utilised by the human body.

Millions of Immune Factors and Growth Factors are transferred into your body, when you take correctly prepared colostrum from a herd of healthy cows.

Immune Factors

The Immune Factors in colostrum comprise six groups of disease-fighting antibodies. These help your body fight off or destroy all types of viral, bacterial, fungal and allergenic invaders.

Colostrum is the only food that provides you with all six groups of Immune Factors that your body requires to effectively fight infections.

The six groups of Immune Factors are as follows:

Immunoglobulins
Leukocytes
Cytokines
Lactoferrin
Interferon
PRP

The following chapters explain these in more detail.

The immunoglobulins in colostrum

The immunoglobulin class of Immune Factors are special proteins carried in the lymph and blood circulatory systems of mammals, including humans. They are the first line of defence in our immune system.

The majority of these immunoglobulins are found in our intestines and are also produced by the intestines.

There are five classes of immunoglobulins. Each beginning with **Ig** and followed by the letters **A, D, E, G** and **M**.

Each class of immunoglobulin has its own unique job to do in the body. This is to attach to, penetrate, destroy, or immobilise a specific type of virus or bacteria.

In a healthy person or animal, there are billions of immunoglobulins. In fact they normally make up just under half of all proteins in the blood.

After a human, or a cow has successfully overcome a disease, it carries an immunity to that disease for many years. Often a lifetime. This immunity is encoded in the immunoglobulin proteins and passed on by females to their offspring.

Human mothers pass on most of this immunity through the placenta, but also through colostrum. Whereas cow immunity is only passed on through colostrum.

This is why cow colostrum has 20 to 40 times more Immune Factors than human colostrum. It is also why a newborn calf normally will not survive without it.

Immunoglobulins are the most important and abundant Immune Factors found in colostrum.

Infections now treated in hospitals with immunoglobulins

Immunoglobulins are now being used in hospitals throughout the world to treat hospital-acquired infections and other diseases.

The *'New England Journal of Medicine'* recently reported that immunoglobulin IgG is so important and effective, that its use has been extended to treat a wide variety of infections and immune disorders, including among many others:

Hepatitis A	Chickenpox	Rheumatoid Arthritis
Multiple Sclerosis	Anaemia	Systemic Lupus
Chronic Fatigue Syndrome		Crohn's' disease

The five classes of immunoglobulins

Below are the five main family groups of immunoglobulins.

IgA A type of immunoglobulin found in the blood, saliva, tears and the mucous of the respiratory and digestive systems. These are the areas of the human body where most invading organisms make their first attack.

IgG The most abundant immunoglobulin found in cow colostrum. It populates the body's lymph and blood circulatory systems where it helps to neutralise bacteria, viruses, toxins and other unwanted invaders. Research shows that IgG can remain in the small intestine and blood stream indefinitely.

IgD A highly effective immunoglobulin virus killer.

IgE Another highly effective immunoglobulin virus killer.

IgM A powerful immunoglobulin bacteria fighter.

The Growth Factors in colostrum

The Growth Factors in colostrum are powerful healing and anti-aging hormones. They regulate the rapid growth of the muscles, bones, nerves and cartilage in the newborn.

Even as adults, they still help us build, retain and repair muscle, bone and nerves.

Growth Factors also help balance blood sugars (to avoid hyperglycaemia and hypoglycaemia), slow down catabolism (the burning of muscle during times of fasting or dieting), and stimulate the burning of fat.

Growth Factors in colostrum are the most widely researched hormones in the world today. Once implanted at birth, they are naturally reproduced by a young and healthy body, but decrease as we age.

Growth Hormone replacement shows outstanding results in slowing down, and even reversing the effects of aging.

Anti-aging clinics around the world can now obtain manufactured copies of certain Growth Hormones. They charge exorbitant fees for something found naturally and in perfect balance in colostrum.

The five Growth Factors in colostrum

Like immunoglobulins, there are also five Growth Factor classes in colostrum.

These five Growth Factors are:

IGF-1 (Insulin-like Growth Factor 1)
EGF (Epidermal Growth Factor)
FGF (Fibroblast Growth Factor)
TGF (Transforming Growth Factor)
GH. (Growth Hormone)

The GF in the code numbers stands for Growth Factor and GH for Growth Hormone.

IGF-1 (Insulin-like Growth Factor 1) This is a complex protein hormone, similar to Insulin and containing 70 different amino acids. It plays an important role in childhood growth and promotes the vigorous growth of youthful cells. It continues to produce muscle growth and bone optimisation even when taken by adult humans or animals.

Almost every cell in the human body is affected by IGF-1, especially muscle, cartilage, bone, liver, kidney, nerve, skin and the lungs. IGF-1 is also believed to cross the blood brain barrier to provide increased mental acuity and increase Serotonin uptake to relieve depression.

EGF (Epidermal Growth Factor) This Growth Factor plays an important role in the regulation, growth and differentiation in the various kinds of body skin cells.

FGF (Fibroblast Growth Factors) This is a complex family of 24 classes, FGF1 to FGF24, These classes all contain sub-families.

They control the growth of new arteries, veins, collagen and connective tissue in the body. FGF is also active in wound healing and the prevention of body defects in growing mammals.

TGF (Transforming Growth Factor) This is another family of hormones, TGF1 to TGF3. They control the forming of and differentiation of various types of body cells. They program the lifespan of these cells and regulate numerous other cell functions.

TGF factors also regulate the immune system killer T cells which help prevent cancer, heart disease and diabetes.

GH (Growth Hormone) This is a highly complex hormone, made up of 191 amino acids, that is stored in, and secreted by our Pituitary Gland. It stimulates body growth and helps to regulate the effects of aging. It can also slow down the effects of aging, and even reverse them to a degree.

Other reported beneficial effects of GH Growth Hormone, seen in adults, include decreased body fat, increased muscle mass, increased bone density, heightened energy levels, improved skin tone and texture and improved immune system function.

Lactoferrin in colostrum

Lactoferrin is one of the most powerful anti-viral and anti-bacterial substances known to man. It is similar to, but even more powerful than the immunoglobulins in its bacteria killing and anti-viral action.

It teams up with the Immune Factor Ig immunoglobulins as our body's first line of defence against a wide range of bacteria, viruses and other microbes.

Lactoferrin is found in mucus secretions, blood, tears, sweat and saliva.

It binds to bacteria and viruses and inactivates them, so that they can then be neutralised by other agents in the body's immune system.

Cow colostrum has by far the highest concentration of Lactoferrin found in any natural food.

Lactoferrin is resistant to stomach acid and able to pass nearly intact into the small intestine, where it operates. From there it is distributed throughout the body as required.

Lactoferrin protects against numerous diseases

Lactoferrin protects the body against a wide variety of health disorders. These include:

- Hepatitis A
- Chicken Pox
- Rheumatoid Arthritis
- Multiple Sclerosis
- Anaemia
- Lupus
- Chronic Fatigue
- Crohn's disease
- Herpes virus

Lactoferrin balances an over-active immune system

Lactoferrin balances the common problem of an over-active immune system, where the body is attacking itself, or is producing too many antibodies.

It also stimulates an under-active immune system.

Lactoferrin has also been shown to play a major role in our body's defence against cancerous tumours. Furthermore, is a powerful antioxidant and is showing promising results with autistic children.

Other Immune Factors in colostrum

Colostrum also contains a powerful blend of many other transferable Immune Factors. Below is a partial list of these powerful Immune Factors, all in perfect combination.

They are solely unique to colostrum and cannot be duplicated in a drug. There are probably more yet to be discovered.

Leukocytes Leukocytes stimulate the production of Interferon, which slows virus reproduction and inhibits the virus's penetration of cell walls.

Lactoperoxidase-thiocyanate, Peroxidase and Xanthine oxidase These three enzymes oxidize (burn up) bacteria by generating the release of hydrogen peroxide.

Lysozyme A powerful immune agent, resistant to acid, that destroys bacteria and viruses on contact. Lysozyme is found in sweat, saliva and tears.

It is now added to infant formulas to boost immune capability.

Cytokines Cytokines regulate the intensity and duration of immune response, and are responsible for cell to cell communications. They boost killer T-cell activity, regulate lymph activity, stimulate production of immunoglobulins and are highly anti-viral and anti-tumorous.

One of the Cytokines, Interlukin-10, is a powerful inflammation inhibitor that significantly reduces inflammation in arthritic joints and other infected or injured areas of the body.

Glycoproteins and Trypsin inhibitors These help prevent the Immune Factors and Growth Factors in colostrum from being digested during their passage through the stomach acid.

They also prevent Helicobactor Pylori bacteria (shown to be the cause of stomach ulcers) from attaching to the stomach wall.

Lymphokines Lymphokines are hormone-like amino acids that help regulate and co-ordinate the immune response in the body.

Oligo polysaccharides, Glycoconjugates, Glycoproteins and Trypsin inhibitors These are various saccharides (sugars) in colostrum. They are attracted to and attach themselves to bacterial invaders, to prevent them from in turn, attaching to or entering the body's mucus-lined membranes.

They are also effective in blocking attachment of Streptococcus Pneumococci bacteria, a major cause of lung inflammation and middle ear infections, E.Coli (the common infected meat bacteria Salmonella), Cryptosporidia, Giardia and Entamoeba (traveller's diarrhea), Toxins A and B and even the highly toxic bacteria that causes diarrhea in cholera.

PRP (Polyproline-rich peptides) PRP peptides, a type of amino acid, are master regulators of the thymus gland, which controls much of our body's immune function.

They are in charge of producing the killer T-cells that fight viruses and pathogens (other toxic substances).

PRP balances an under-active or over-active immune system, where the body is actually attacking itself. This disorder gives rise to the diseases of Multiple Sclerosis (MS), Rheumatoid Arthritis, Lupus, Sclera Derma, as well as common food and environment allergies.

Prolactin, Insulin and Glycoproteins These also help protect the many Immune Factors and Growth Factors in colostrum from being destroyed by stomach acid and other digestive enzymes.

Why colostrum from dairy cows?

Obtaining colostrum from humans is simply not practical.

Human mothers are not always healthy, or free from substance addiction. And not many would want to give up their life-giving colostrum.

Requirements for colostrum to be safe and viable

It is therefore necessary to look to an animal source. There are a number of requirements for animal colostrum to be safe and viable:

- The Immune Factors and Growth Factors must be biologically transferable to humans.
- The collection must come from a large pool of animals, in order to provide broad-based Immune Factors.
- It must be a commercially viable source, that assures a hygienic and plentiful gathering process.

Dairy cows are the only animals that meet all of this criteria.

Advantages of cow colostrum

Bovine (cow) colostrum is accepted by virtually all mammals, including humans. Interestingly, no other animal but the cow is able to be a universal donor and have its Immune and Growth Factors transferable to humans.

In the USA and Japan, researchers have verified, in laboratory analysis, that the Growth Factors (IGF and TGF) and the key Immune Factors (immunoglobulins) in cows, are identical in molecular structure to humans and are not species specific.

In other words, they are fully transferable from one species to another.

Further research has shown that colostrum from cows is much richer in Immune Factors than colostrum from humans.

Human colostrum contains only 2% of IgG, the human body's most important immunoglobulin, compared to cow's colostrum which contains around 20% IgG.

Colostrum transfer factors can survive stomach acid

Many might assume that colostrum, when taken via the stomach, would be digested by the stomach acid, like any other protein.

But scientists proved in clinical research back in 1975, and again in 1994 that cow's colostrum contains special inhibitors of Glycoproteins, Trypsin and Protease.

These shut down the stomach acid and digestive enzymes that normally digest proteins such as immunoglobulins and Growth Factors, allowing them to remain active as they pass into the small intestine.

Colostrum however must be taken on an empty stomach, allowing at least 30 minutes before a meal, as other food can override this shutting down of digestive enzymes and acids.

It is also important to note that these digestive inhibitors are only present in cow colostrum during the first 24 hours after birth. It is important that colostrum only be gathered during this brief time.

This is one of the major reasons that Immune Factors found in dairy whey are not effective in human use. They are in fact digested by the body for fuel.

A doctor L. B. Khazenson carried out a study on human volunteers in which cow colostrum was taken orally. Samples taken from their digestive tracts proved that the important immunoglobulins survived the passage through the stomach and were effective in providing protection.

This and a significant number of other human trials from the 1950's through to present times, have proven that the digestive route for immune protection by colostrum works.

The history of colostrum use

Historically, cow colostrum has played a significant role in natural healing. It has been used in India for thousands of years. Ayurvedic physicians have documented colostrum's health-giving benefits.

They even make a candy by dropping colostrum in boiling water and then coating it with sugar.

Northern European countries

People in Scandinavian and northern European countries are also familiar with the healing benefits of colostrum. To celebrate the birth of a calf and their own good health, they make a delicious colostrum dessert, topped with honey.

In the US and throughout the world, cow colostrum was used for antibiotic purposes prior to the introduction of antibiotics.

In the early 1950's, colostrum was prescribed extensively for treating the inflammation of Rheumatoid Arthritis.

Provided the antibodies for polio vaccine

In 1950, Doctor Albert Sabin, famous for the polio vaccine, was aware of the possibilities of colostrum. He found that bovine colostrum contained antibodies for polio (even though cows don't appear to get polio). He refined these antibodies, growing them in a cultured media and produced the world's first anti-viral vaccine.

Thousands of clinical trials world-wide show colostrum is safe and effective

Hundreds of years of human use, and thousands of scientific studies and human clinical trials world-wide, have shown bovine colostrum to be safe and effective.

Colostrum's rediscovery and the extensive subsequent research, show that we have had one of the most important supplements for immune enhancement and body tissue repair available all along.

Processing colostrum for maximum effectiveness

For maximum effectiveness, colostrum should come from cows that are antibiotic and hormone free.

It is also important that colostrum be standardised by taking it from a large number of healthy cows. This insures the maximum possible quantity of Immune Factors.

Colostrum that is not standardised is hardly worth taking.

Manipulating Ig percentage can diminish effectiveness

Some colostrum is manipulated by processors to boost the immunoglobulin (Ig) levels. Recent research however, has shown that higher percentages of immunoglobulin can actually diminish colostrum's effectiveness in combating infection.

The most effective colostrum is that which is gently processed, but otherwise left with the balance of its Immune and Growth Factors as Nature intended.

Predominantly pasture-fed cows best

Where possible, try and find colostrum that comes from predominantly pasture-fed herds.

When a cow eats healthy, green grass, it gets the live enzymes that it is naturally designed to eat, and its colostrum contains more of these beneficial enzymes. This helps make the benefits of colostrum more readily available for humans.

Colostrum should be water-soluble to gain the full benefits

Research has shown that colostrum which is water-soluble is more easily assimilated. If you are taking colostrum which is only partially soluble, you may not be getting the full benefits.

With capsules, you can check solubility by simply emptying a capsule into a glass of water. It should dissolve quickly when stirred.

Excessive heat destroys biological activity

Tests on several different brands of colostrum have shown that colostrum processed with excessive heat will lose most of its biological activity.

Powder generally better than tablets

This is especially true of colostrum tablets. The heat generated when tablets are formed can be so high as to severely compromise colostrum's value.

Not all colostrum processed in accordance with strict guidelines

Currently no standards are enforced for the collection and processing of colostrum. Some colostrum contains inexpensive 'filler' products such as whey by-products, which severely reduce its efficacy.

Needs to be collected during first 24 hours

Unless colostrum is collected during the first 24 hours after the birth of the calf, it will be missing many of the important Growth and Immune Factors.

Liposomal delivery to ensure full bio-availability

Within two days after birth, our human digestive system begins functioning. From this point on, some of colostrum's vital factors can be digested and no longer have any effect.

Fortunately there is natural protection against moderate stomach acid built into colostrum. But this can be easily overridden if taken with food, especially high fat foods, which require a strong concentration of hydrochloric acid in the stomach to digest them.

This is why it is necessary to take colostrum on an empty stomach for it to be effective.

Modern research has however found a way to provide more protection from the body's digestive system than is naturally provided by colostrum, so as to better insure that all of the Immune Factors and Growth Factors are available to the body.

The method to achieve this is called liposomal delivery. During processing, the colostrum molecules are coated with tiny globules of fatty membranes, which help insulate the molecules from digestive acid in our stomach.

This does of course make this type of colostrum more expensive. It should however be remembered that regularly processed colostrum has always given excellent results when taken with water on an empty stomach.

10 standards for highest quality colostrum

To help you assess different brands of colostrum, here is a summary of the standards you should look for in high quality colostrum.

1. It should be fully water-soluble and never frozen.

2. If should come only from certified healthy, Grade A dairy cows (after the needs of the calf are met).

3. It should be collected only from the first two milkings after the second birth, to ensure maximum biological activity.

4. It should come only from cows which are predominantly pasture-fed, and certified to be antibiotic and hormone free.

5. It should only be flash pasteurised, to ensure the highest microbiological activity is retained.

6. It should be mixed with the colostrum from thousands of other cows, to standardise and maximise the billions of Immune Factors.

7. Unwanted fat should be removed during processing and the colostrum dried without added heat. (This process is more costly and time-consuming than regular, high-temperature processing.

8. It should be certified laboratory tested for absence of E.Coli, salmonella, heavy metals, antibiotics, pesticides and other harmful substances.

9. It should be certified laboratory tested for high platelet count, a sign of active, friendly intestinal microflora and Immunoglobin (antibody) content.

10. Most importantly, the colostrum should be gathered and processed by a dairy company that is certified by an appropriate government agency, for example the United States Department of Agriculture. Companies should show proof of this certification on their label or in their literature.

There are not many producers of bovine colostrum which meet the above high standards. So read labels carefully and investigate the company.

Bear in mind also, that much colostrum is processed for the veterinary industry and not intended for human consumption.

Independent research organisations
Another way to find a high-quality colostrum is to contact an independent research organisation such as the Center for Nutritional Research (CNR), Sedona, Arizona. www.icnr.org.

CNR can provide, free of charge by email, a list of processors whose colostrum meets their guidelines.

Conditions that allow disease to develop

The onset of almost all infections and degenerative disease is preceded by a suppressed immune system. Our body's immune system is designed to recognise and destroy disease-producing agents.

Factors that suppress our immune system

There are four major factors that suppress or lower our body's immune system:

Genetic We inherit genetic strengths and weaknesses from our parents. Genetic weaknesses can allow disease to develop if conditions are right.

Lifestyle An unhealthy lifestyle can wreak havoc on our immune system. We suppress our immune system with nutritional deficiencies, a sedentary life, overwork, stress and exposure to toxins.

Toxins Toxins in the environment have never been at a higher level. Their effect on our health can be critical, so wherever possible we must minimise our exposure to them.

Nutrition We are fortunately becoming more aware of how important it is to meet our body's nutritional requirements. To balance the intake of protein, carbohydrate, fats, vitamins and minerals.

Lack of antioxidants

Today, we hear a great deal about the importance of antioxidants in maintaining our health.

A deficiency of Vitamin A (an antioxidant) can actually shrink the thymus gland, limiting killer T-cell production. Killer T-cells are our major line of defence against microbe attack.

Vitamin E and other antioxidants protect Vitamin A from becoming ineffective through oxidation.

Vitamin C is a powerful antioxidant and effective in fighting infection. Vitamin C also protects water-soluble nutrients from oxidation, by being oxidised itself.

Lack of protein

Protein is vital to maintaining a healthy immune system. Essential amino acids, found in animal proteins, need to be balanced with the non-essential proteins from plant sources.

Protein helps maintain a steady blood glucose level in the body, and is critical for brain function.

Lack of Vitamin B12

Researchers have recently discovered that Vitamin B12 can actually double the body's immune capabilities. Therefore, because of the importance of trace nutrients such as Vitamin B12, and their inter-dependence upon each other, we must eat a well balanced diet.

If we choose a diet that is lacking in even one nutrient that our body requires, we need to supplement that nutrient in our diet.

Accumulation of toxic wastes

Nutritional deficiencies also impair that part of our immune system, designed to rid our body of the toxic waste that accumulates in our cells and tissue.

This provides an open invitation for the scavengers of nature, bacteria and viruses, to come along and feed on the dying tissue.

Lack of exercise

Without adequate aerobic and weight-bearing exercise, our body does not function well for long.

A sedentary lifestyle accelerates our aging process, depresses our immune system, slows our metabolism, causes us to gain weight, weakens our heart muscle and decreases our mental acuity.

We should set aside time to exercise each day and make this an important priority.

Stress and overwork

If stress and overwork appear to be unavoidable, we need to take an honest look at our priorities.

Aging

The last factor is aging. As we age, our ability to fight infection and disease decreases.

Our society places much emphasis on the superficial aspects of aging; plastic surgery, hair implants, wrinkle creams, liposuction, etc.

These procedures would be unnecessary if our bodies retained the fully active hormonal balance, cell repair and immune systems of our youth.

What if there was a supplement that restored these systems, giving us increased longevity?

We would value this supplement even more, if it improved our quality of life by slowing down, or possibly reversing our outward aging signs, and gave us more energy and zest for living.

We would also appreciate our bodies burning fat, our muscles toning up quickly, elasticity returning to our skin and our body healing faster.

As you learn more about colostrum, ask yourself, is it possible there is a fountain of youth after all?

Organisms that cause infectious disease

Disease-causing organisms, from microscopic viruses, bacteria and fungi, to larger parasites are found in soil, on plants, in animals and in food.

Although these organisms can produce disease, they are normally kept under control by our immune system. If our system is weak, or we encounter an organism to which we have not built up an antibody resistance, illness can result.

These disease-causing organisms are as follows:

Viruses: In its simplest form, a virus is just a strand of DNA or RNA, surrounded by a bit of protein. It is too small to be seen, even through a light-operated microscope. Its presence is detected only from the boiling or bubbling of the cells that have been invaded.

A virus cannot reproduce on its own, as can bacteria. Viruses only reproduce and mature within a cell's interior cytoplasm (cytoplasm is the material from which cells are made). Viruses actually use body cells as tiny factories to reproduce more of their own kind.

When they mature, the viruses explode the cell's wall, destroying the host cell and infecting nearby tissue. The cycle is repeated and the disease spreads.

Flu and the common cold, Hepatitis, Chronic Fatigue syndrome, Polio and AIDS are a few of the viral diseases.

Bacteria: These are round or rod-shaped, microscopic one-cell organisms. They live without the need for other organisms, and are able to multiply by sub-division.

When infectious bacteria enter the body, they multiply and produce powerful chemicals (toxins) that can damage the cells in the tissue they have invaded.

Some of the more common classes of bacteria that cause disease are Staphylococci, Streptococci, Chlamydia, Haemophilus, Gonococci and Rickettsia.

Fungi: Moulds and yeasts are fungi, but only certain moulds and yeasts are infectious.

Candida albicans is one virulent example. It produces thrush (infection of the mouth and throat) in people who have received antibiotics, or have impaired immunity.

It also infects the bowel, robbing the body of essential nutrients and can lead to leaky gut syndrome.

Protozoa: Protozoa are single-cell organisms that live within the body, usually in the intestinal tract as a small parasite. Most are harmless, although some, like malaria can cause disease.

Helminths: These are large parasites that take up residence in the intestinal tract, lungs, liver, skin and even the brain. The most common Helminths are tapeworms and roundworms.

Our first lines of defence against disease

The immune system of our body has many mechanisms to defend against infectious organisms. The medical term for an infectious organism is 'pathogen'.

Our skin, respiratory system (nose, mouth, throat and lungs) and gastro-intestinal tract (stomach and intestines) provide the first lines of defence against pathogens.

If pathogens get past these first three barriers, the immune system takes up the challenge of eliminating the invaders.

To do this, our immune system employs both physical and chemical defences.

The skin

Our skin acts as a protective barrier to bacteria, viruses, parasites, toxins and other pathogens.

If our skin is broken, pathogens such as staphylococci bacteria can enter our body and start an infection. Damp skin, especially in warm climates, attracts various types of bacteria and fungus.

However the skin's acidity, along with sebum from the skin's oil glands, discourage many bacteria and micro-organisms.

Perspiration also contains Lysozyme, an enzyme that destroys bacteria by eating through the bacteria cell wall. This enzyme is also found in nasal fluids, saliva, tears and tissue fluids. It destroys viruses as well as bacteria.

Mucus and hair-like cilia

Mucus-coated nasal hairs trap pathogens and pollutants from the air we breathe.

Cilia (hair-like projections) guard our upper respiratory tract. They move pathogens and dust that become trapped in the mucus lining of the bronchioles (branches of the lungs) toward the throat. Here they are swallowed, or expelled as phlegm.

Sneezing and coughing also help us get rid of mucus-trapped pathogens.

The membranes (soft inner body skin) that line the nasal and respiratory passages, the digestive tract, the colon and the urinary tract are also lined with mucus. However these mucus-lined membranes are not as strong or reliable at keeping out invaders as our outer skin.

Because the membranes are warm, and coated with a liquid mucus to keep them from drying out, this invites micro-organisms who thrive in warm moist conditions. When enough of them gather, they can break through a membrane.

Injury or irritation to our membranes can also be caused by the toxic waste of micro-organisms. This too can allow a break-through.

Viruses are so small, they can travel through the tiny passages in the digestive tract membranes designed for food absorption.

The lower bowel, which is the most polluted part of the human body, is the main entrance for pathogens and toxins to invade the body. The mucus lining of the bowel, while providing a barrier to disease, is a breeding ground for harmful bacteria and unhealthy flora.

Stomach acid

Stomach acid (hydrochloric acid) destroys most bacteria and their toxic wastes.

However, it still allows some friendly lactobacillus acidophilus (acid loving) bacteria to pass into the small intestine, where they help us process nutrients and protect our bowel.

Our second line
of defence –
immune response

If infectious agents (pathogens) break through our first lines of defence, to attack our body and gain control of our vital cells and organs, our body mobilises the second line of defence. This protection is known as the immune response.

So when an pathogen breaks through our outer skin or mucus barrier inside our body, whether it is a bacterium, virus or toxin, it quickly comes across the main defenders of our body called leukocytes, more commonly known as white blood cells.

There are different kinds of these leukocytes, or white blood cells, and they can multiply very quickly in times of infection. That is why a raised white blood cell count usually means there is an infection present.

The circulatory passages of our body's blood and lymphatic systems carry these leukocytes and their chemical messengers to the sites of infection.

There are two main types of leukocytes comprising these white blood cells, antibodies (immunoglobulins) and killer T-Cells.

The antibody (immunoglobulin) defence

Our antibody immunity is made up of antibody proteins called immunoglobulins. These are normally manufactured by our white blood cells in response to a foreign substance (a pathogen). Or they can be supplied from colostrum. These antibodies circulate in our blood and other body fluids.

Generally any foreign substance (or pathogen) that enters the body, either through our digestive system, a wound, or by injection, will cause the manufacture of an antibody. It neutralises the pathogen or renders it harmless.

The antibody so produced only fits the unique protein surface pattern of the pathogen and that alone.

Once an antibody has been formed, the pathogen it matches is called an antigen. The antibody fits the antigen like a key fits a lock. The antibody, which is a small bit of protein, smaller than bacteria. It sticks to the antigen like glue and cannot be shaken off.

After the antibody locks onto the antigen, it changes shape, to attract another special protein found in our blood, which in turn releases a chemical that penetrates the cell wall of the foreign antigen and kills it.

Antibodies are only effective against the antigen that caused its creation. Colostrum contains innumerable antibodies. These antibodies combine with the ones already present in our immune system.

An example of how our bodies create antibodies, to protect our health, is found in the science of immunisation. A toxin that has been rendered harmless to your body, but is still capable of producing an immune response, is injected into the body. The body recognises the toxin and responds by creating antibodies that will neutralise the toxic substance.

These antibodies begin to circulate in the body's fluids and usually persist for many years.

Even when they have finally disappeared, as your body has learned how to manufacture a particular antibody, it can resume production of that antibody quite rapidly. This is why a vaccine booster shot is sometimes recommended in later years, to again stimulate the production of protective amounts of these antibodies.

Killer cell (leukocyte) immunity

Killer T-cells in our immune system (called leukocytes), along with their associated helper cells and suppressor cells, are specialised white blood cells. Killer T-cells originate in our thymus gland or bone marrow and are boosted and activated by colostrum.

There are different types of killer T-cells, and they assist each other to protect or kill body cells that are under attack from infectious pathogens such as viruses, fungi and cancer.

The eight main types are as follows, each with a specific function:

Main killer T-cells These are white blood cells, derived from the thymus gland which is the master control gland of the immune system. They seek out, lock onto, and destroy body cells that have been infected by an invading pathogen. They do this by releasing a chemical poison.

Helper killer T-cells These increase the number of killer T-cells that can engulf or dissolve infected cells in response to an attack.

Suppressor killer T-cells These help avoid over-production of killer T-cells and suppress them when necessary.

Natural killer Lymphocytes (NK) These are specialised 'green beret' like forces that patrol the body, killing virus infected cells.

These natural killers also play a major role in destroying cancer cells. Small numbers of cancer cells are constantly being destroyed in the body by these lymphocytes. It is only when conditions are unfavourable for defence, such as high acidity, that cancer cells increase.

Phagocytes (scavengers) There are two classes of phagocytes. Those that ingest bacteria, and those that ingest infected particles, dead tissue and defective or aged cells.

Mediator cells These carry helper cells that slow blood flow and widen blood vessels to aid the fighter cells movement into battle.

Lymphocytes These are aggressive cells that have two key roles. They directly kill infected cells by releasing a poison, or they resort to chemical warfare by releasing other substances to produce required immune responses.

Lymphocytes are found in the bone marrow, in the spleen, circulating in the blood and in the lymph nodes.

The lymph nodes are collections of lymphocytes, held together by connective, fibrous tissue. Lymph nodes are located in the neck, groin and armpits where they can be felt if they become firm and enlarged in the course of a disease or infection.

Other lymph nodes are found in the tonsils, abdomen and at the centre of the lungs.

Lymph is a colourless fluid that runs in channels from all parts of the body, through the lymph nodes and ultimately back into the bloodstream. The lymph nodes create a filter for harmful organisms that may be travelling in the lymph. These cells grab and destroy these pathogens as they pass by.

Some lymphocytes energetically hunt for virus-infected cells in the blood and lymph circulatory systems. When they find one, they puncture a hole in the cell membrane, allowing the inner cytoplasm to leak out, which eventually kills the cell.

Infectious organisms also have complex offensive systems

So as we see, the body's immune system is a complex defence system for suppressing and eliminating infections.

However, at the same time, infectious organisms have their own complex offensive systems. The result is a constant battle between your body and disease. A battle your body usually wins, but not forever.

But colostrum significantly improves the odds.

Colostrum as a natural antibiotic

Research centres world-wide that are looking seriously at the natural process of immunity, are putting much of their focus on colostrum. They are continually discovering new and important components in colostrum.

No more potent antibiotics left

After 50 years of aggressive antibiotic abuse, doctors are now confronting bacteria that have evolved defences against these drugs. Patients are succumbing to once easily treatable infections.

Even with the 30 or so antibiotics that drug companies claim to be working on, there appear to be no more potent antibiotics left to treat these drug-resistant bacteria.

Also, animals are being fed antibiotic-laced feeds or are given regular injections, in an effort by commercial producers to ensure their maximum growth and survival until they reach market.

Without antibiotics, the chicken, beef, pork and lamb that you buy would not be so plentiful, and would therefore be much more expensive.

But the problem is, that when we consume these meats, we get residuals of the antibiotics that the animal has been fed or injected with, and so our bodies become desensitised to their constant presence. When we really do need an antibiotic, more and more powerful varieties are required to do the job.

There may be only one solution to protect ourselves against antibiotic-resistant bacteria, and that is colostrum. With its natural Immune Factors that stimulate and increase the natural capability of our immune system.

Colostrum increases the supply of antibodies and activates killer T-cells

Colostrum's primary benefit is in building the body's own immune system, so it can function with strength all on its own.

Colostrum increases our supply of antibodies and primes the production of our body's own antibodies.

Furthermore, it boosts and activates the killer T-cells in our blood, that identify and destroy viruses and infected cells.

Other ways colostrum heals your body

Colostrum provides its most powerful benefits in the areas where nearly 80% of all disease and infections enter the body – the mucus-lined surfaces of the airways, lungs and intestinal tract.

Most infectious diseases that enter the body, remain localised on mucosal surfaces.

Peyer's Patches

The largest mucus membrane of the body is the intestinal tract, followed by the lungs.

There are special lymph node areas in the intestines and lungs known as Peyer's Patches (named after their discoverer Swiss anatomist Johann Peyer).

There are about 30 patches in the body, each about 40mm long and 10mm wide. They produce antibodies to destroy disease on our mucus membranes and also in our circulatory system.

Over 70% of our antibodies are produced by the Peyer's Patches in our intestines. So it is obvious that we should focus in this area if we are serious about preventing disease. Infections in the intestines can lead to infections in the lungs. Most of the antibodies in colostrum remain in the intestinal tract after being swallowed.

These antibodies in colostrum, stimulate the production of more antibodies at the Peyer's Patches in the intestines and lungs. They are then sent throughout the body where they coat and protect tissue and destroy pathogens, toxins and allergens.

Antibiotics make our immune system vulnerable by destroying beneficial bacteria

In recent years, a flood of antibiotics, antihistamines and food preservatives have seriously unbalanced, diminished or destroyed the beneficial bacteria in our small intestine. (Our small intestine is actually about 7 metres long and contains about a kilogram of bacteria).

This has hampered our immune systems, making them less effective and allowing virulent bacteria to take over.

With repeated antibiotic use, our immune function is further lowered. This can result in new food and environmental allergies that have never troubled us previously.

Even when antibiotics are stopped, the immune system is weak and vulnerable until it builds up strength again.

There is only so much toxicity our intestines can handle before our lungs and airways are affected also. Asthma often then becomes a problem.

In large numbers of people, the toxic overload nowadays is so great, that normal defences and healthy useful bacteria are at the point of being overwhelmed.

Hard-training athletes more susceptible to infectious

Studies also show that an exhaustive workout is followed by a temporary immune depression, with a marked decrease in the number of infection-fighting killer T-cells.

These changes can last for several hours. As a result, some hard-training athletes develop long lasting debilitating conditions, similar to chronic fatigue syndrome.

Studies with animals further confirm that exhaustive exercise increases the risk and severity of infections.

Fortunately, colostrum's numerous Immune Factors result in a major reduction in infections caused by physical stress.

Colostrum promotes healthy intestinal microflora

Colostrum also has the proven ability to promote healthy intestinal microflora, as the friendly bacteria in colostrum can find its way into the small intestine without being destroyed by stomach acid.

Colostrum not only promotes healthy intestinal microflora, increasing nutrient absorption, but it fights disease, reduces gas and bloating and stops leaky gut syndrome.

How colostrum stops leaky gut syndrome

The contents of our lower bowel contain a toxic waste mixture from which the body needs to be protected.

How the body protects itself from bowel waste

Protection from bowel waste is normally provided by a mucus barrier on the inner bowel lining.

Any toxins that penetrate the gut wall, are removed by being engulfed by immunoglobulins, or oxidised by the actions of specialised amino acids and proteins found in the bile.

However the cost of this detoxification is high. It consumes large amounts of antioxidants.

Any harmful substance that escapes these twin defences and passes into the bloodstream, must then pass through a third defence, the liver, which filters them out of the bloodstream.

Numerous diseases caused by a leaky gut

A leaky gut is caused by permeability of the intestine wall, or an ineffective mucus barrier. This often causes diarrhea and other diseases. It also creates allergies to certain food substances, and even allergies to normal bowel flora.

In experiments with animals, it has been shown to produce auto-immune disorders where the body's immune system attacks healthy body tissue.

Diseases associated with increased intestinal permeability, called leaky gut syndrome are numerous. To name just a few:

Acne
Autism
Chemical sensitivities
Cholera
Chronic Arthritis
Chronic Fatigue Syndrome
Crohn's disease
Cystic Fibrosis
Dermatitis
Diarrhea
Environmental hyper-sensitivity
Hepatitis
Hyperactivity

Infectious Enterocolitis
Inflammatory Bowel disease
Irritable Bowel Syndrome
Pancreatitis
Psoriasis
Salmonella and E.Coli infections

Causes of a leaky gut

Leaky gut syndrome is usually caused by exposure to infectious agents such as bacteria (E.Coli), viruses (rotavirus), yeasts (candida), intestinal parasites and various toxins.

Additional causes are alcoholic beverages, anti-inflammatory drugs, high levels of free radicals (food borne or produced by inflammatory cells), toxic drugs, reactions from heart attack, surgeries or shock.

The relationship of a leaky gut to food allergies can begin early in life, with even infants reacting to allergens in their food.

Colostrum and continued breast feeding will normally prevent intestinal permeability. Colostrum can prevent the onset of leaky gut syndrome, diabetes and allergies.

Nutritional absorption hindered

Intestinal wall disorders will also generally disrupt nutritional absorption. Malnutrition then occurs, which further hinders cell repair and immune functions. This in turn causes infections, disease and bowel permeability to worsen.

Safe, non-invasive means to test for leaky gut

Leaky gut syndrome often goes unrecognised. However there are safe, non-invasive means to test for intestinal permeability.

Colostrum can stop leaky gut syndrome

Colostrum can stop leaky gut syndrome. Its immunoglobulins IgA, IgG and IgM, Lactoferrin and other Immune Factors stop the reproduction and penetration of bacteria and toxins.

The Growth Factors in colostrum stimulate repair of the intestinal barrier. Its anti-inflammatory action reduces cellular spacing, stopping permeability.

Nutritional deficiencies need to be corrected

To allow the rebuilding of immune functions, there is usually the need to correct nutritional deficiencies, such as the addition of more fibre for proper bowel passage.

Also the elimination of known allergenic foods (at least temporarily) and toxic oral drugs and antibiotics.

Protection against cholera and candida

Human clinical trials have shown that colostrum is able to neutralise not only bacteria and viruses, but also their toxins. Even toxins from the deadly bacterial family that includes tetanus and botulism.

There are also several dangerous varieties of the common E.Coli bacteria found in the bowel. These can cause diarrhea and are highly irritating to the bowel because of their toxic metabolic wastes. Research has shown that colostrum is effective against this type of E.Coli bacteria, by preventing its growth and neutralising its highly toxic wastes.

Cholera protection

Both IgA and IgG immunoglobulin antibodies in colostrum can provide protection against cholera. At Ohio State Children's' Hospital, colostrum from cows exposed to cholera, and thereby containing antibodies to the disease, protected children against contracting cholera.

Candida controlled

Candida albicans (yeast) infections usually occur after the use of antibiotics. When this infection invades the digestive system, healthy microflora (intestinal bacteria) are overcome by unhealthy bacteria. Nutrient absorption becomes restricted and the immune system is severely weakened.

A study by the University of Hong Kong showed leukocytes (white blood cells) in colostrum were effective in controlling the candida infection.

Lactobacillus Acidophilus and Lactoferrin which are present in colostrum, are also powerful agents against this destructive intruder.

Allergies and auto-immune diseases controlled by PRP in colostrum

Allergies and auto-immune diseases such as multiple sclerosis (MS), rheumatoid arthritis, lupus, pernicious anemia, and myasthenia gravis are caused by an over-reaction of the immune system. Too many antibodies are produced in response to an attack by an pathogen (toxic substance).

Allergies and auto-immune diseases are a medical dilemma. The body's healing mechanism becomes too powerful and begins destroying health by attacking healthy joint cells, or nerve and skin tissue.

Fortunately this over-active immune response can be toned down with one of the most powerful components in colostrum, PRP (Proline-rich polypeptides).

PRP in colostrum offers enormous possibilities

Researchers in Poland studying colostrum discovered PRP (an immune-regulating amino acid). They found that PRP was non-species specific, in other words PRP in cow's colostrum will benefit humans.

PRP assists the body's thymus gland in balancing the immune system, especially where the immune system is over-active and killer T-cells are attacking the person's own body.

This appears to be the case in rheumatoid arthritis, multiple sclerosis (MS), A.L.S., lupus, sclera derma and food and environment allergies.

Out-of-control killer T-cells can create enormous inflammation, discomfort and debilitating pain as they destroy the body's connective joints and skin and nerve tissue.

PRP inhibits the over-production of killer T-cells and other lymphocytes, which have been stimulated by pathogens. It stops the progress of the attack, reduces the associated pain and swelling and can return the body's immune balance to normal.

Viruses destroyed

Colostrum is the only food that will destroy viruses. Something no other food or drug can yet do.

This is why colostrum has been shown to be effective in stopping colds, cold sores, flu viruses, viral bronchitis, viral pneumonia, herpes, and chronic fatigue syndrome.

What is a virus?

A virus is nothing more than a little piece of RNA.

RNA is an enzyme-like strand, carrying a computer-like code, found inside living cells with the role of instructing the thousands of DNA genes within the cell, as to which of them are to be activated and when.

Viruses move about the world, looking for compatible places to hide and grow. They are practically indestructible and can retain their capabilities to reproduce for days, even years in harsh conditions that would kill bacteria.

Viruses need an animal or human cell to replicate

Viruses have one thing in common, they need animal or human cells to replicate themselves. Therefore in order to combat them, we must either stop them before they enter a new cell and begin to multiply. Or kill them after they have entered, by destroying the entire cell in which they live.

Colostrum contains a wide range of effective anti-virus Immune Factors, Immunoglobulins, Lactoferrin, Leukocyte stimulators, Cytokines, etc.

The ever mutating HIV virus

Antibodies (immunoglobulins) and white blood cells (leukocytes) kill most viruses, but they can't stop the fast mutating HIV virus. This attacks the immune system itself and can lead on to the usually fatal AIDS disease.

The virus mutates so quickly that the immune system is unable to produce antibodies and killer T-cells quickly enough to cope and is eventually overcome.

The final result is that an AIDS patient comes down with other opportunistic infections, both bacterial and viral that the immune system is no longer capable of handling, as it is too busy and weakened from fighting the HIV virus.

However Immune Factors in colostrum have shown their unique ability to help, even with this rapacious killer. Colostrum has been proven in numerous clinical and human trials to be effective with the opportunistic infections, even when virtually all other treatments have failed.

Diarrhea is a major reason why AIDS patients' immunity becomes compromised. Chronic diarrhea not only reduces the ability to fight infections (75% of the body's antibodies are produced by the intestinal immune system) but it also drains the body of vital nutrients, electrolytes and body fluids.

Lactoferrin, another bacteria-fighting protein found in colostrum also inhibits the growth of HIV, by preventing penetration of the body cells.

The cause of gross weight loss and muscle wasting

A human body, without proper nutrition, and under stress, produces cortisol, which causes catabolisation (eating its own muscle for energy).

Cortisol is highly suppressive to our immune system, so an already severely weakened immune system is further suppressed.

The effects of this process can be seen in the gross weight loss and muscle wasting so evident with this terrible disease.

Colostrum is the key to keeping the gut pathogen-free and functioning optimally.

Hyper-immune colostrum

Hospital clinical tests have experimented with hyper-immune colostrum and found it to be highly successful.

Hyper-immune colostrum is produced by injecting a healthy pregnant cow, with a specific virus or bacteria. The cow then produces the specific Immune Factors for that particular invader.

Colostrum is then collected from the cow after birth of her calf and fed to patients with the specific virus or bacteria.

Interestingly however, double blind human trials have found that hyper-immune colostrum is only 15% more effective in these circumstances, than regular cow colostrum (67% versus 82%).

Hyper-immune colostrum is understandably in short supply and only generally available under hospital supervision.

How colostrum can prevent a heart attack

Many cardiac (heart) diseases are the result of immune over-sensitisation to damaged heart muscle.

Heart muscle dies after it is damaged in a myocardial infarction (heart attack). The body then produces antibodies to dispose of these new pathogens (particles of dead heart muscle).

If these antibodies become over-active, they produce an inflammation condition in good heart muscle, similar to an auto-immune response. This often results in a further heart attack.

PRP in colostrum, with its ability to regulate over-active immune functions, plus the other anti-inflammatory factors in colostrum, can lower the risk of additional heart attack.

Colostrum promotes regeneration of heart muscle

Growth Factors in colostrum have the unique ability to promote the healing and regeneration of heart muscle tissue and new blood vessels. These factors are significant in the acceleration of recovery.

Bacteria linked to formation of plaque in arteries

Research has also found that a common type of Chlamydia bacteria is linked to the formation of plaque in the artery walls of about 80% percent of patients with heart disease.

LDL/HDL cholesterol balance improved by colostrum

IGF-1 and GH, in colostrum, have been shown to lower LDL cholesterol concentration (a sign of higher heart attack risk) and increase HDL cholesterol concentrations (a sign of reduced heart attack risk).

Cancer and colostrum

Cancer has many causes, but in great part is due to cell damage from a genetic predisposition for toxic build-up in cells, and cell acidity, which nearly all cancer invaded cells require to survive.

Viruses also seek out toxic, acidic or damaged cells to enter for replication. The older we get, the more damaged cells we have.

However colostrum provides an impressive mix of Immune and Growth Factors that limit and inhibit the growth of cancer cells.

Cytokines to boost Killer T-cell activity

Colostrum contains other Immune Factors known Interleukins 1, 6 and 10, Interferon G and Lymphokines. These are called Cytokines.

Cytokines boost killer T-cell activity and stimulate production of other immunoglobulins. They are highly anti-viral and anti-tumorous. Cytokines are one of the most researched factors in the search for cancer cures.

Lactalbumin can cause suicide of cancer cells

Additional Immune Factors in colostrum help in other ways. Research doctors in Sweden found that colostrum contained Lactalbumin, a substance found to have the unique ability to cause cancer cell apitosis (suicide), leaving surrounding cells untouched.

Growth Factor, Growth Hormone and Lactoferrin also fight cancer

Growth Factor TgF-B in colostrum has been found to have cytoxic effects (kills them) on human bone cancer cells. It also inhibits the growth of bone cancer cells (a 75% reduction), is highly anti-inflammatory, repairs tissue and promotes the healing and formation of bones.

Experiments also show that the presence of cancer cells stimulates a reaction of Growth Hormone in colostrum that mobilises large numbers of Leukocytes to come and engulf the cancer cells.

Also Lactoferrin, a major component of colostrum, has unique abilities to fight cancer and other disease.

Reducing the side effects of chemotherapy and radiation treatment with colostrum

Chemotherapy and radiation severely compromise the immune system, putting patients in grave danger from infection, especially from within the intestinal area.

One of the most devastating symptoms of gastro-intestinal infections is chronic diarrhea, which depletes the body of water, electrolytes and other life-supporting nutrients.

Cortisol (the stress hormone) is then produced, signalling the body to live off stored nutrients. However this normally suppresses the immune system.

Colostrum is able to halt this destructive process, restore nutritional absorption and rebuild resistance and strength.

Colostrum is desperately needed to survive most of the orthodox treatments prescribed for treating cancer today.

Diabetes and colostrum

Cause of Type 1 diabetes

Type 1 diabetes is currently thought to result from an over-active immune system, attacking and damaging the pancreas gland, resulting in a lack of insulin output. This allergic reaction is believed to arise due to the protein GAD, found in cow's milk.

This reaction has been shown to occur in children who did not receive human colostrum, or a long enough course of breast feeding. Colostrum and human mother's milk contains factors that can offset an allergy to GAD.

In fact colostrum helps offset all allergic reactions in our body.

IGF-1 in colostrum an
effective alternative to insulin

(Insulin) Growth Factors IGF-1 in colostrum, bond with the Insulin Growth Factor receptors found on all cells in the body.

Growth Factor IGF-1 blood levels in diabetics have been found to be lower than in non-diabetics.

Therefore Growth Factor IGF-1 can be an effective alternative to insulin in normalising glucose transport in diabetics.

Causes of Type II diabetes

Type II diabetes is directly related to lack of exercise, lack of Growth Factor IGF-1 and poor nutrition.

With Type II diabetes, there is also increased risk of heart disease, stroke and hyperglycemia (high blood sugar). IGF-1 alone is an effective treatment for acute hyperglycemia.

Growth Factor IGF-1 essential for weight loss

Without IGF-1 our bodies will not burn fat

Both Growth Hormone GH and Growth Factor IGF-1 shift calorie burning from carbohydrate to fat.

In fact without the presence of Growth Factor IGF-1 in our body, we will not burn fat. This is a major reason for stubborn obesity.

As IGF-1 is essential in processing fat to burn for energy, lack of it means that our body burns blood sugar and protein as the main fuels for energy. This protein burning appears to have the effect of lowering IGF-1 body levels still further.

So without IGF-1, during times of extreme exercise, or when fasting or extreme dieting, instead of burning its fat stores, the body simply burns its own protein and blood sugar.

Colostrum spares protein during exercise

However, sports researchers have found that with an elevated level of IGF-1 in the body, the rate of catabolism (body muscle protein being burned for energy) following an exhausting work out is decreased. Even under conditions of protein deprivation.

Less efficient fast-twitch muscle fibre increased in body with lack of exercise

Sports research has also found that in circumstances of lowered physical activity, the percentage of lower efficiency, fast-twitch muscle fibre increases in the body.

This type of muscle does not burn calories as efficiently as low-twitch muscle.

Importance of exercise IGF-1 and nutrition for weight reduction and body condition

If we expect to reduce our weight and improve our body condition, it is important that both aerobic and weight resistant exercise be done. Also our Growth Factor IGF-1 levels and proper nutrition intake must be maintained.

Normally our body will produce sufficient Growth Factor IGF-1 if we are taking care of it and eating a balanced nutritional diet.

But a significant reduction in Growth Factor IGF-1 will be caused by lack of exercise, improper nutrient intake, exposure to toxins and normal aging.

Colostrum better than steroids for muscle growth

Growth Factor IGF-1 promotes muscle growth. It speeds up protein manufacture and as we saw in the last chapter, reduces or stops protein catabolism (protein burning by the body for energy).

This leads to an increase in lean muscle mass, without a corresponding rise in fat tissue.

A prominent body building researcher, Daniel Shawn reported in an article in Ironman Magazine (a magazine for serious body builders) in 1992: *"There is no other compound in the universe, to date, which can help you better than IGF-1. Not steroids, not bio-technology and genetically engineered GH Growth Hormone, not Releasing Factors, not even a strict diet of pure amino acid and glycogen. Plain and simple, IGF-1 is the end all, and the be-all of anabolic peptide growth factors"*.

New muscle cell growth

University of Arizona researchers have further confirmed, that when Growth Hormone GH, Growth Factor IGF-1, Transforming Growth Factor TgF-A and Epithelial Growth Factor EgF are administered in combination, they can stimulate new muscle cell growth.

The muscle cells, so stimulated, fuse with adjacent muscle fibre, increasing the total number of muscle cells.

Does our body create Growth Factor?

Our body does create and maintain a level of Growth Factor naturally, but this steadily reduces with age and lack of exercise.

Normally we can only increase Growth Factor IGF-1 in our body naturally via colostrum.

Can Growth Factor IGF-1 be commercially manufactured?

Growth Factor IGF-1 can be manufactured commercially (using yeast and E.Coli bacteria), but it has proven to have dangerous, diabetic-like side effects in the body.

Rapid healing

The healing and regenerative effects of colostrum extend to nearly all the structural cells of our body.

Growth Factor IGF-1, Transforming Growth Factor TgF-A, Growth Hormone GH, and Epithelial Growth Factor EgF (which promotes normal skin growth) are all useful for muscle, nerve, bone, skin, and cartilage repair.

The factors above can also speed up wound and surgery recovery, and stimulate the rapid healing of ulcers.

Topical skin and gum healing

Colostrum is excellent for topical (skin) healing. Epithelial Growth Factors EgF in particular, stimulate skin growth and regeneration.

Colostrum can be applied directly to minor cuts, abrasions and burns that have first been cleaned and disinfected.

Powdered colostrum can also be applied directly to gums in cases of gingivitis, sensitive teeth and mouth sores with excellent results.

Both internally and externally, colostrum heals, protects and builds.

The fountain
of youth

The New England Journal of Medicine, the most prestigious Medical Journal in the world, reported that the most effective way to stop or slow the aging process, would be to regularly renew the hormones that regulate normal cell reproduction in the body.

After age 18, the level of Growth Hormone that our body naturally produces, begins to dwindle. We eventually notice this as gravity, unmercifully takes its toll.

Our bodies lose muscle tone and skin elasticity, causing us to sag and wrinkle. We also lose bone mass and shrink, making our hands, feet, nose and ears look larger.

Colostrum safely increases muscle mass and strength in the aged

There is an answer. A natural answer. Colostrum's perfectly balanced combination of Immune and Growth Factors.

When administered in human clinical trials with aged subjects, colostrum safely increased Growth Factor IGF-1 to pre-puberty levels, producing increased muscle mass and strength.

Growth Factor IGF-1 and Growth Hormone GH in colostrum have also been shown to tone muscles, melt off body fat, return elasticity to the skin and increase bone density.

Colostrum, life's first food, has given those who are growing old, real hope that there may be a Fountain of Youth after all.

Colostrum can stimulate the growth and repair of DNA

Everything in life springs forth from DNA – flesh, bones, hormones, nervous system, a baby's first word. The euphoria that comes with first love. The ability to learn a foreign language. All of this originates from DNA.

DNA attracts the chemicals it needs to form new DNA. This is an essential part of cell division.

DNA is also able to manufacture RNA, the 'instruction software' of DNA. RNA is nearly identical to DNA and provides the active intelligence to produce the proteins needed to build and repair the body.

Dr. Benjamin Frank in his research on youth and aging, showed RNA to be one of our most critical anti-aging factors. His research showed that the Growth Factor IGF-1, found naturally in colostrum is one of the only substances known, to stimulate the growth and repair of these genetic code carriers.

Japanese researchers further discovered that Transforming Growth Factor TgF even promotes the repair of DNA when it has been damaged. It also suppresses production of abnormal cells.

Colostrum is unique, in all the world for its ability to support our body's basic intelligence, DNA and RNA.

Stimulation of sexual response

Other anti-aging factors found in colostrum are Gonadotropin-releasing hormone (GnRH), and its amino acid (GAP). Both of these stimulate sexual response.

Colostrum can enhance mental acuity
and brighten our moods

Furthermore, Growth Factor IGF-1 and Growth Hormone GH, some of the smallest particles known, have been shown to cross the blood brain barrier, to help with nerve synapses in the brain.

The effect is to enhance mental acuity, and increase serotonin levels to brighten our moods.

Colostrum has also been shown to help maintain blood glucose levels to serve the brain optimally.

As we age, this might be one of the most important reasons to take a serious look at colostrum.

How to use colostrum effectively

Bovine colostrum is safe, non-toxic and can be consumed in any quantity, without side-effects or any known drug interactions.

It contains enzymes that protect its Immune Factors and Growth Factors from being destroyed by stomach acid, or digested. It should however be taken only on an empty stomach with water.

Safe for internal consumption by children, adults and animals

Robert Preston, ND, President of the International Institute of Nutritional Research, states, *"Bovine colostrum is safe. Colostrum contains an unprecedented combination of nutritional factors with which to fortify the immune system. It is so harmless, it has been prepared by Nature as the first food for infants, intended as their total diet for the first 24 hours. It would be hard to imagine any nutritional substance more natural or beneficial than colostrum. It is safe for internal consumption by children, adults and animals."*

How much do I take?

You should take enough colostrum to obtain results. <u>If you're not seeing results with colostrum, you are probably not taking enough.</u>

Adults should begin with a minimum of 3000mg per day, (approx 3 slightly raised teaspoons) or six 00 size capsules).

It can then be lessened to a maintenance level of about 1500mg a day, as long as it continues to produce results.

Take on an empty stomach

Colostrum has a 16 hour half life, therefore it should be taken twice a day on an empty stomach, with a glass of water.

If taking it as a powder, dissolve the powder first in the bottom of a glass by stirring it with a small amount of water to a smooth runny paste. Then add the rest of the water, usually half to a full medium size glass. The amount of water is not critical.

If the colostrum is difficult to dissolve, warm water can help. But not so warm that you cannot comfortably immerse a finger in it. Otherwise the active factors may be harmed by the heat.

Dissolvable colostrum is better absorbed.

How long does it take to feel the benefits?

Colostrum's benefits are cumulative. The longer and more

consistent you use it, the greater the benefits. Most people feel better right away. Some go through a rough 'healing crisis' reporting flu-like symptoms such as fatigue, nausea, diarrhea, headache, coughing up phlegm, skin rashes and low grade fever.

This usually lasts only a few days. The body is ridding itself of long-accumulated toxins that have been locked up in the body's tissues and fat deposits. These have probably suppressed your immune system and encouraged disease.

<u>Do not decrease use at this time. In fact, it is probably a good time to temporarily increase the amount you take.</u>

Most people with disease are feeling so bad anyway, that the knowledge that their body is healing will pull them through any difficult initial period.

Can babies and children benefit too?

Colostrum is not just for adults. There are often remarkable results with babies and children.

Colostrum's proof is in the undeniable superior health of children who received colostrum and breast milk from their mothers. Research consistently shows that these children experience less illness, increased mental acuity and have stronger, more vibrant growth.

Unfortunately, mothers sometimes face circumstances where it is not possible for them to provide their children with this wonderful natural food.

Newborns and premature babies who did not get colostrum, can greatly benefit from the bovine source, but this should be done under medical supervision.

Children's age and weight should to be considered when giving them colostrum. Start with half the adult amount. However no harm has been reported from higher amounts than this.

Continual use of colostrum for children is generally unnecessary, since they soon naturally produce within their bodies most of colostrum's active factors.

So its use with children after an initial course, can be held for those times when colds, flu, viral or bacteria invasion or disease may be lessened with its use. Or when antibiotics or drugs may have compromised their body's immune functions.

Appears to be even more effective on animals

We should not forget our pets. Veterinary use of bovine colostrum with aging or ailing mammals has proven to be highly beneficial. Its ability to stop disease is well documented. It appears to be even more effective than with humans.

Conclusion

Colostrum is renowned for its powerful healing factors. It gives us a natural and safe answer for optimal health.

Medical research, presented by doctors and scientists from hospitals and universities around the world, state that the presence of such a wide spectrum of immunoglobulins, antibodies and other Immune Factors, found in colostrum, offer tremendous benefit in the prevention of and recovery from illness.

Colostrum's Immune Factors have been found to not only boost the underactive immune system, but to regulate an over-active immune system which causes allergies and auto-immune disease.

Colostrum's Growth Factors promote tissue repair, with many regenerative and anti-aging benefits.

These Growth Factors also help build muscle, burn fat for energy, build and repair RNA and DNA, increase uptake of blood sugar, and regenerate nerve, skin, bone and cartilage tissue.

Colostrum's great potential to fight disease, improve quality of life, and increase longevity is unprecedented.

It can not be duplicated in a scientific laboratory. Its unique combination of Immune and Growth Factors are only possible from nature. Colostrum is life's first food and it is perfect.

Colostrum is perfectly safe

It is always important, whenever you are impressed by claims and testimonials that a health product will benefit you, that you make certain there is supporting research for these claims. And that you can have confidence the product will not harm you in any way, create harmful side-effects, or conflict with any medical drug or other supplement you may be taking.

In this regard, colostrum, which is a food, has been proven to be safe, non toxic, non allergenic and have no side effects.

Colostrum testimonials

Reports from people using bovine colostrum cover a huge range of health benefits and near miraculous cures.

Most commonly are heard the following:

- Weight loss.
- Feelings of well-being.
- Dramatic reductions and elimination of pain and disease.
- Accelerated healing after surgery, wounds and broken bones.
- Elimination of colds and flu.
- Increased physical strength and endurance.

Here are just a few excerpts from heartfelt stories that keep pouring in.

All Multiple Sclerosis (MS) symptoms have left my body

"I feel like I have truly found a miracle in my life. I have suffered from multiple sclerosis for seven years. After taking colostrum for only a couple of months (three teaspoons a day) all MS symptoms have left my body (dizziness, weakness and fatigue, eye problems, burning sensation in my feet). I am able to walk without a limp and climb stairs without the aid of a railing. I cannot say enough good things about this miraculous food."   Bonnie; Ogden, Utah.

Improvement in energy level, better sleep, relief from muscle aches and pains

"My doctor's diagnosis was that I had Epstein Barr Virus and he recommended a six month disability. After taking colostrum for a month I found a notable improvement in my energy level, an ability to sleep, relief from muscle aches and pains and I was able to begin exercising. I am recommending colostrum to all of my friends and family."   Natalie; Salt Lake City, Utah.

Severe burn healed without scarring

"I severely burned my wrist on an engine block. I was told that it would take at least a month to heal and would probably leave an ugly scar. With colostrum it was completely healed without scarring in one week."   Howard; Bethesda, Maryland.

Polymyalgia and depression healed

"I was diagnosed with Polymyalgia Rheumatica. Colostrum has not only helped me physically, but also mentally and spiritually. I am no longer depressed because I am getting better and better. My husband appreciates the 'new me'. I would recommend colostrum very highly for those who want the finest quality of life."

Rhoda; Clearwater, Florida.

Severe depression lifted, only 10 days to heal from knee replacement surgery, flatter stomach, lower blood pressure

"I am a 70 year old man who this last year has gone through a devastating personal experience that led to severe depression. For ten months, my doctor prescribed numerous anti-depressant drugs that didn't help at all. After taking colostrum for two months, my depression lifted."

"I also had a total knee replacement two weeks ago. I had the other knee replaced a year ago and it took forever to heal. To everyone's disbelief, ten days after my surgery I was out dancing."

"My muscles are more defined and my stomach is noticeably flatter."

"My blood pressure has dropped from 145/85 to 120/70 and my pulse has gone from 83 to 70. I have been able to come off heart medication."

Bill; Holladay, Utah.

Itchy skin problem for years, healed in days

"I have had hives internally and externally that even the strongest medication hasn't helped. Within days of taking colostrum, 95% of my symptoms were gone. For the first time in years, I am able to wear clothes comfortably, sleep, go to work, eat normal foods and cuddle with my wife."

"I have more energy and I'm less moody. My wife thinks she's married a new man. I have my life back, plain and simple. There are no words to express how incredible this is and what it means to me."

Warren; Murray, Utah

Painful bursitis in both my hips gone

"I have been troubled with very painful bursitis in both of my hips for the last three years. Night time was the worst, because any movement would waken me to pain. I have had physical therapy treatments regularly to obtain some relief. Because I was so miserable I decided to try the colostrum. At first, I didn't think that it was helping me, but after three weeks I was pain free. I have always been quite a skeptic, so I was truly surprised and very happy."

Janet; Cottonwood, Utah.

Stronger muscles, rapid healing after surgery, no flu

"*Years ago I broke my right shoulder twice and my left shoulder once. With any lifting I would dislocate my shoulders. Colostrum has given me noticeable upper muscular strength and I no longer have a problem with lifting.*"

"*I had arthroscopic knee surgery shortly after I started taking colostrum. They had to smooth the knee cap and repair cartilage. I was back at work and climbing stairs two hours after surgery.*"

"*My work brings me in close contact with over forty men on a daily basis. I am the only one that hasn't been sick this winter. I've never felt better and I guess it shows, because everyone tells me that I look better than I have for years.*" Ken; Salt Lake City, Utah.

I lost 3½ inches off my waist

"*Since having breast cancer in 1991, I've had a difficult time losing weight. After only one month of taking colostrum, I lost seven pounds, 3½ inches off my waist, and an inch off my bust and hips.*"
Georgia; Fairbanks, Alaska.

Blurry vision cleared up in one week

"*I was getting worried because my eyes wouldn't focus for distance after reading the newspaper (everything was blurry). Day by day this problem seemed to get worse. Thank God for colostrum. It cleared up the problem in one week.*" Judy; Sandy, Utah.

Red inflamed eyelids completely cleared

"*I was diagnosed with Blepharitis (inflammation of the eyelids). Areas on my face became red, swollen and itched. Steroid creams did not help., But with colostrum, my problem has completely cleared up.*" Pat; Salt Lake City, Utah

I can now eat anything I please, and no more flu

"*I've taken colostrum for just one month and my stomach and intestinal tract has never felt better. No more bloating and indigestion. Now I can eat anything I darn well please. I've noticed that the flu bug that everyone is getting is passing me by.*"
Robert; Salt Lake City, Utah.

Vision improved, gums stopped bleeding, more energy, muscles firmer, hair thicker, fingernails grow faster

"*Because of colostrum, my vision has improved, my memory seems better, my gums have stopped bleeding, I have more energy and my muscles are firmer. It's as though I've been working out at the gym for months. For the first time, my allergies are 90% better.*

I just can't believe it when I look in the mirror. I look like I've had a facelift. Incredible! My fingernails and hair are healthy (thicker and grows faster). Colostrum is truly a miracle in my life. I am so grateful!"   Deanna; Palmer, Alaska.

No more warts
"Nothing would touch my warts. If they were removed, more would come back in their place. After taking colostrum, I have no more warts."   Jimko; Germany (age 11).

Slimmer waist, bigger chest, less wrinkles, age spots disappeared, colds and flu gone in an hour
"I've taken two inches off my waist and increased my chest 1½ inches after two months of taking colostrum. My skin is softer, with less noticeable wrinkles. My age spots have disappeared. If I feel a cold or flu coming on, I take a big spoonful of colostrum and the symptoms are gone in an hour."   Alan; Holladay, Utah.

95% of my symptoms of Multiple Sclerosis gone
"I suffer from Multiple Sclerosis. On the regular dose of colostrum, I noticed that I felt stronger and my fatigue was easing up. I increased my dose and after one month, 95% of my symptoms are gone. Incredible difference."   Lisa; Ashley, Pennsylvania.

Sinus problem cleared, more energy, more cheerful, a cold healed in two hours
"For the last three years, I have suffered from sinus pain. Colostrum cleared my sinuses. I ran out and the problem was back. I started the colostrum again and will not go off of it again."

"Besides relief from sinus pain, colostrum keeps me from going into the doldrums, gives me constant energy and an overall sense of well-being. My brother thought that he was coming down with a cold on two occasions. A couple of hours after taking colostrum, he felt great."   Kirk; Holladay, Utah.

Diabetic blood sugar levels dramatically improved
"I am a non- insulin diabetic. I've been taking colostrum for just over a month. I went to my doctor for my routine tests. My blood sugar levels had dramatically improved for the first time. This colostrum really works."   Pete; Holladay, Utah

Now able to eat solid foods again
"I haven't been able to eat solid foods for three years because I have advanced Sclera Derma (a debilitating auto-immune skin

disease). *All nourishment had to be taken in liquid form. After just one week of taking colostrum, I was able to go out to dinner with my family and eat a whole hamburger. There are no words to express what colostrum means for myself and my family."*

Sydney; Concord, California.

Psoriasis completely cleared up

"I've had Psoriasis for 23 years. It covered my stomach and buttocks and legs. Since taking your American Colostrum back in December 2008, it has completely cleared up and has not come back." David; Motueka; New Zealand.

Chest lifted back up

"I have been taking colostrum the last three months, and since then, with no additional exercise, my 63 year old chest appears to have lifted back up to where it was when I was much younger."

David; Tauranga, New Zealand.

Age spots not as brown

"I have finished my first lot of colostrum. The age spots are not as brown as they were." Peter; Papatoetoe, New Zealand.

Impotent no longer

"My husband age 72 was beginning to suffer from impotency, but no longer. I am very appreciative." Pauline; Auckland, New Zealand.

Cancer shrunk, no more colds, life back

"I have had cancer of my immune system in the abdominal area since 2000. I have done chemo's and stem cell transplants. When I read about colostrum I thought, 'There is nothing to lose in trying this product out.'

"To me it is the greatest product on the market. My cancer has shrunk. I don't get colds, and mainly it has given me my life back. I fully recommend this product. My doctors have said, "Whatever you are doing, just keep doing it."

Wiesia; Mt Maunganui, New Zealand.

Stomach pains gone after 10 years

"After 10 years of continuous stomach pains, I tried one 500ml jar of powdered colostrum. I took a level teaspoon, five times a day in a ¼ glass of milk. After three weeks the pain went and has not come back." Denis; Te Kuiti, New Zealand.

What doctors say about colostrum

Concentration of a lifetime's immunity

"When a (mammal) ... gives birth to its offspring, its mammary glands filter out of the blood the immune factors it has acquired through a lifetime of fighting disease-causing organisms. It then concentrates these factors into special non-milk, immune supporting fluid called colostrum. A mother animal produces true colostrum for only the first twenty-four hours after giving birth."

Robert Preston. MD. President, International Institute of Nutritional Research.

Inhibits stomach ulcers, reduces arthritis inflammation

"Glycoproteins, in bovine colostrum, inhibit the attachment of the Helicobactor Pylon bacteria that cause stomach ulcers. Colostrum contains significant amounts of Interlukin-1 0, found significant in reducing inflammation in arthritic joints and injury areas."

Dr. Olle Hemell. University of Ulmea, Sweden.

"Colostrum contains Glycoprotein that protects against the bacteria that cause stomach ulcers." **Dr. Raloff.** Science News.

Colostrum neutralises the most harmful bacteria, viruses

"Immunoglobulins (found in colostrum) *are able to neutralise the most harmful bacteria, viruses, and yeasts."* **Dr. Per Brandtzaeg.**
Annals of the New York Academy of Sciences.

Effective against disease-causing organisms in the intestinal tract

"Immune factors in cow colostrum, when taken orally, are effective against disease-causing organisms in the intestinal tract." (Results of human clinical study.) **Dr. R. McClead**. Pediatrics Research.

Colostrum regulates allergies

"Clinical studies show that IgE (immunoglobulin) found in bovine colostrum, may be responsible for regulating allergic response."

Vastly beneficial to aged and immuno-deficient

"Colostrum stimulates the lymphoid tissue providing benefits in aged or immuno-deficient people. Oral administration of immuno-factors is simple, inexpensive, free of side effects and may be vastly beneficial in veterinary and human medicine, to correct immunodeficiency."
Drs. Bocci, Bremen, Corradeschi, Luzzi & Paulesu. Journal Biology.

Prevents viral and bacterial infections

"Immunoglobulin from bovine colostrum effectively reduces and prevents viral and bacterial infections in immune deficient subjects; bone marrow recipients, premature babies, AIDS, etc." New England Journal of Medicine

Anemia, Multiple Sclerosis, Lupus, Rheumatoid Arthritis, Chronic Fatigue, Crohn's disease all successfully treated

"Immunoglobulin in colostrum has been used to successfully treat: Thrombocytopenia, Anemia, Neutropenia, Myasthenia Gravis, Guillain Barre Syndrome, Multiple Sclerosis, Systemic Lupus, Rheumatoid Arthritis, Bulluos Pamphigoid, Kawasaki's Syndrome, Chronic Fatigue Syndrome and Crohn's disease, among others."
Dr. Dwyer. New England Journal of Medicine.

Activates an underactive immune system, suppresses an over-active immune system

"PRP in bovine colostrum, has the same ability to regulate activity of the immune system as hormones of the Thymus gland. It activates an underactive immune system, helping it move into action against disease-causing organisms. PRP also suppresses an over-active immune system, such as is often seen in the auto-immune diseases."
Dr. Staroscik. Molecular Immunology.

"Turns white blood cells into functionally active T cells. Results were shown in treatment of auto-immune disorders and cancer. An important immune modulator, stimulates an underactive immune system and tones down an over-active one." **Drs. Janusz & Lisowski.** Immunology.

75% inhibition of bone cancer, healing of heart muscle

"Bovine colostrum contains TgF-B which has an important suppressive effect on cytoxic substances. Inhibits cell growth of human osteosarcoma (bone cancer) *cells (75% inhibition). Mediator of fibrosis and angiogenesis* (healing of heart muscle and blood vessels)." **Dr. Tokuyama**
Cancer Research Inst. Kanazawa University. Japan.

Stimulates cartilage repair

"Cartilage-inducing Factor, found in colostrum, stimulates cartilage repair." **Drs. Seyedin, Thompson, Bentz.** Jnl. of Biological Chemistry.

Colostrum accelerates wound healing

"Growth factors in bovine colostrum were found to be very effective in promoting wound healing. Recommended for trauma and surgical healing. External and internal applications." **Dr Sporn.** Science.

"Accelerated healing is possible for treatment with trauma and surgical wounds." **Dr. Bhora.** Journal Surgical. Restoration.

DNA restoration

"Bovine colostrum contains high levels of growth factors that promote normal cell growth and DNA synthesis (restoration).*"* **Drs. Oda & Shinnichi.** Comparative Biochemical Physiology.

Stimulates nerve regeneration

"IGF-1 found in colostrum, stimulates bone and muscle growth and nerve regeneration." **Drs. Skottner, Arrhenius-Nyberg, Kanje & Fryldund.** Acta. Paediatric Scandinavia, Sweden.

Increased muscle growth in aged

"High age is associated with reduced levels of growth hormones. Induction of GH and IGF-1 increase body weight through muscle growth of aged subjects." **Drs. Ullman, Sommerland & Skottner.** Dept. of Pathology and Pharmacology, University of Gothenburg, Sweden.

Fat burning increased by 50% and increased energy

"GH (Growth Hormone) inhibited the insulin stimulated glucose disposal by 27%, and raised non-protein energy expenditures. Fat oxidation contributed 71.7% of energy expenditures during GH administration, as compared with 48% without. Conclusion: GH increases energy expenditures and inhibits glucose oxidation in favour of increased lipid (fat) *oxidation* (burning).*"* **Bak, Moller, Schmitz** University Clinic of Internal Medicine, Aahus Kommunehospital, Denmark.

Inhibits burning of body muscle for energy

"IGF-1 inhibits malnutrition-induced catabolism (stops the burning of body *muscle* for energy.)*"* **Gluckman, Breir and O'Sullivan.** Department of Pediatrics, University of Auckland, New Zealand.

What researchers have discovered about colostrum

Colostrum 21 times richer in Vitamin B12 than regular milk

Dr. Samson and associates found colostrum was 21 times richer in Vitamin B12 than milk. Adequate B12 in body doubles the body's immune systems ability to fight disease.

Dr R. R. Samson. *Immunology.* Vol 38, No 2, pp291-296.

90% of calves die without colostrum

Calves without colostrum die in 90% of cases. Feeding commercially prepared colostrum can provide immediate compensation. **Berl & Munch.**
Bovine Colostrum and Protection of Young Animals, 105 (7), p219-24.

Immunity factors from cow colostrum transferable to humans

Immune regulatory factors in bovine colostrum are transferable to human and other species. **Watson, Fransis & Ballard.**
Journal of Diary Research, (3, pp369-80.

Dr. Khazenson completed a study on human volunteers in which cow colostrum was taken orally. Samples of their digestive tract demonstrated that the immune factors were effective in providing protection, prevention and treatment of acute intestinal diseases. **Dr Khazenson.**
Microbial and Epidemial Immunobiology, No 9, pp101-106.

Cow colostrum has a phenomenal 40 times more effectiveness than human colostrum

Dr. Bruce demonstrates that human colostrum contains only 2% IgG (the body's most important immunoglobulin) while cow colostrum contained a phenomenally more, up to 40 times that amount. **Dr C. E. Bruce.** *Natural History,* Feb 1969.

Colostrum perfectly safe

Colostrum found to be perfectly safe. No known contradictions or overdoses. **R. Preston.** *International Institute of Nutritional Research. "Bovine Colostrum. Human consumption."*

Colostrum not affected by stomach acid

A special glycoprotein in cow colostrum is effective at protecting the immune and growth factors in colostrum from destruction by digestive acids in the human stomach.   **A. Pineo.**
Biochemical Biophysiology Acta, (Amsterdam) 379, pp201-206.

Protease inhibitors in colostrum shut down digestive enzymes that normally digest proteins, allowing them to remain active as they pass into the bowel.   **Von Fellenberg & Hoeber.**
Schweiz. Arch. Tierheilkd, Vol. 122, No 3, pp159-168.

Reduces arthritis inflammation

Colostrum contains significant amounts of Interlukin-10, a strong inflammation inhibitory agent significant in reducing inflammation in arthritic joints and injury areas. **Hernell & Olle.**
University of Ulmea, Sweden. *Science,* Apr 1995, pp 231.

Blocked major cause of ear infections

Colostrum blocked attachment of Streptococcus Pneumococci, a major cause of middle ear infections.   **Hanson.**
Annals of New York Academy of Sciences, p409.

Colostrum protects the area most diseases attack

Most infectious diseases attack the body through the mucus surfaces of the intestinal tract. This is where colostrum does most of its work.   **Waldman.**
Annals of New York Academic Science, Vol. 409, pp510-515.

Mucosal surfaces produce 70% of our body's antibodies. The mucosal system is therefore the most important area to concentrate attention in prevention of disease.   **Service.**
Science, v265, pp1522-1524.

Immunity from cholera passed onto babies by mother's colostrum

Mothers in India, exposed to cholera, passed on protective antibodies to their newborn which prevented them from getting the disease.   **Majundar.**
Infection and Immunology, Vol. 36, No 3, pp962-965.

Numerous powerful antioxidants

Colostrum was found to contain numerous powerful, naturally occurring, antioxidants.   **Buescher, Mcllheran.**
Pediatric Research, Vol. 24, No 1, pp14-19.

Protection from numerous common disorders

Colostrum provided antibodies to the bacteria, viruses and yeasts responsible for the following conditions: appendicitis, meningitis, bronchitis, pneumonia, candida albicans, chicken pox, cholera, diarrhea, dysentery, diphtheria, gastroenteritis, encephalitis, respiratory infections, pneumonia, polio, septicemia (blood poisoning), tetanus, typhoid, myelitis, and whooping cough." **Ogra, Lesonsky & Fishout.**
Research. State University of New York at Buffalo.

Colostrum effective against E.Coli and Candida

Mother sheep and cows given doses of E.Coli orally, developed antibodies in their colostrum. When nursing offspring were then dosed with E.Coli, immune factors from the mothers' colostrum prevented the E.Coli from attaching to the bowel wall and protection resulted. **J. A. Morris.**
Journal of Medical Microbiology. Vol. 13, No 2, pp265-271.

Colostrum prevents or slows virus growth

Colostrum stimulated production of interferon, the substance that slows or prevents viral growth. **Lawton.**
Archives of Disease in Childhood, 54, pp127-130.

Colostrum from cows exposed to cholera, contained antibodies which protected against that type of cholera in offspring.
Richard McClead. *Pediatric Research,* Vol. 6, No 4, p227.

Bronchitis and pneumonia immunity
passed on through colostrum

Animals exposed to the RSV virus, often responsible for bronchitis and pneumonia, passed on antibodies against this virus in their colostrum. **Christine Theodore.**
'Immunologic Aspects of Colostrum and Milk. Raven Press, NY.

Immunity from bowel inflammation and diarrhea

Japanese researchers exposed cattle to rotavirus, which causes severe diarrhea and bowel inflammation in humans. Colostrum from these cows contained antibodies which, when fed to humans, prevented them from getting rotavirus.
Ebina. *The Lancet,* Vol. 29, No 2, pp1029-1030.

Prevention of diarrhea among travellers

Colostrum protects against shigellosis (digestive upset) and may be useful in preventing diarrhea among overseas travellers.

Jacket, Binion & Bostwick.
American Journal of Tropical Medicine, Vol 47(3), pp276-83.

Colostrum contains all key immunoglobulins

Confirmation that bovine (cow) colostrum contains all four key immunoglobulins, and that they are not species specific. **Harper.**
Review of Physiology Chemistry, Lang Medical Publ, Los Gatos, CA.

DNA repair

Japanese researchers discovered that Transforming Growth Factors A and B (TgF A & B) in colostrum promoted the synthesis and repair of DNA, the master code of the cell.

Noda. *Gann,* Vol. 75, pp109-112.

Bovine (cow) IGF-1 identical to human IGF-1

Analysis of Growth Factor 1, IGF-1, from bovine colostrum found it to be to be identical to human IGF-1.

Francis. *Biochemical Journal,* 233(1), pp207-213.

Colostrum Growth Hormone restored
muscle tissue and power in old rats

Administration of growth hormone to old rats, raised the level of IGF-1 to that of young rats. This restored the muscle protein manufacture of the old rats. They grew more muscle tissue and the muscle had increased maximum contraction force.   **Ullman.**
Acta Physiol Scand, v140, pp521-525

Remission of diabetes in mice with colostrum

Diabetic mice treated with the colostrum resumed normal regulation of their blood sugar and kept free of the disease.

Science News, Vol 145, p37

Cancer cell destruction

Colostrum Transforming Growth Factor produced cell destruction in human cancer (sarcoma) cells in cell culture growth experiments in Japan. **Toluyama.** Cancer Research Inst.
Kananawa University, Japan. *Cellular Biology Report 13*, pp251-258.

A-lactalbumin (from colostrum) caused lung cancer cells to create selective suicide (apoptosis). Normal surrounding cells unaffected.   **Hakansson.** *Proceedings.* Nation Academy of Sciences.
Lund University, Stockholm, Sweden, Vol. 92, pp8064-8068.

About the authors

Daniel G. Clark, M.D.

Dr. Clark received his Doctorate of Medicine from the Medical College of Georgia. In 1984 he was awarded the *"Academic Award for Scientific Research in Cancer"* (Academia Internationale Di Pontzen) in Rome, Italy. He received the *"Physician of the Year"* award in Broward County, Florida in 1988.

He is founder of company, BioActive Nutritional, Inc., Melbourne, Florida and has been actively involved with numerous professional associations and teaching centres. Dr Clark sponsors educational seminars for physicians worldwide, providing lectures on quantum and molecular medicine. Recently he was invited as keynote speaker on Anti-Aging at an international conference in the Republic of China.

His special interests are in the study of aging and health therapies for arteriosclerosis, alternative treatments for cancer, and homeopathy and herbology for the prevention and treatment of chronic disease.

Kaye Wyatt

Kaye Wyatt is a retired teacher who has currently dedicated herself to informing people everywhere of the benefits of colostrum. This commitment arose out of her own healing experience with this amazing superfood. See her story on page 6.

Kaye's new career as a writer was a direct outgrowth of her commitment to spread the word about colostrum. It has led to appearances on national radio, television, and at health-oriented expositions.

She currently lives in Sedona, Arizona with her husband, Douglas Wyatt, who is Director of the Center for Nutritional Research, which specialise in research on colostrum

David Coory

David Coory who has edited and revised this updated edition of the book, is a New Zealand nutritional researcher and author.

He is the author of New Zealand's top selling nutrition book for the past 15 years *"Stay Healthy by Supplying What's Lacking in Your Diet"*. He has also authored, edited and co-authored other books, mostly on health.

He currently resides in Tauranga, New Zealand.

Made in the USA
Middletown, DE
06 December 2015